DEADLY DISEASES:
An Inside Look

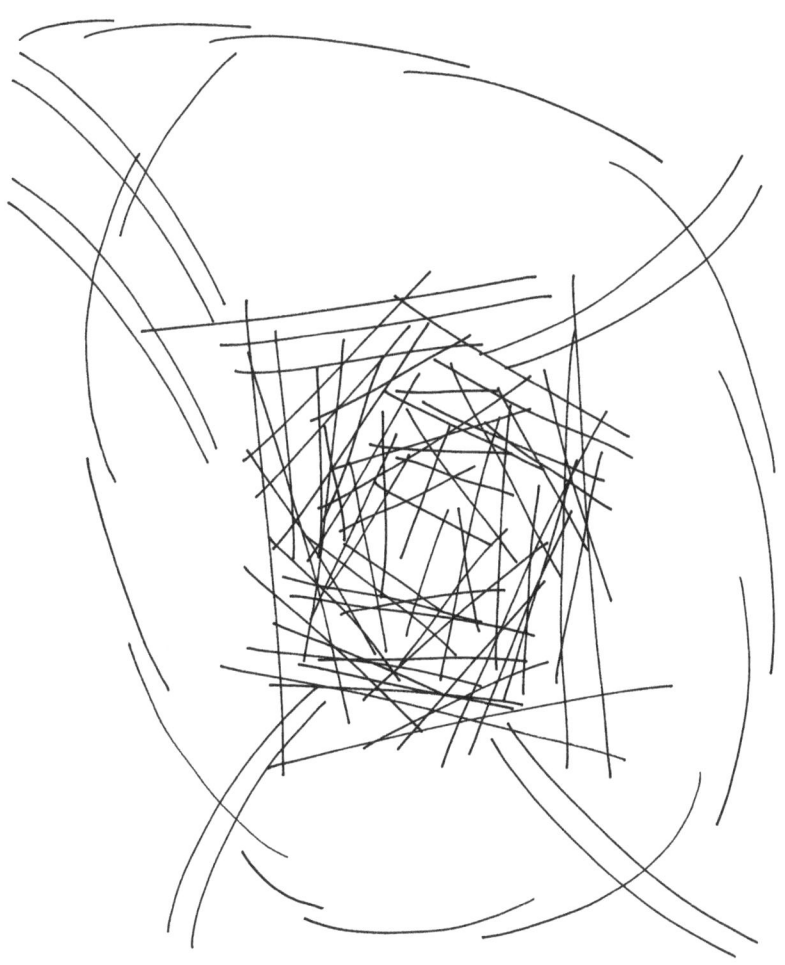

Camilia MacPherson, Ph.D., D.Th.
2016

INTRODUCTION

This book is written using Automatic Drawings and Surreal Art in the style of Scholars' Art. There is no top or bottom to the page. Each page should be viewed from every angle and varying depths. The pre-calligraphy graphics as seen in the diagram below indicates the complexity of these markings.

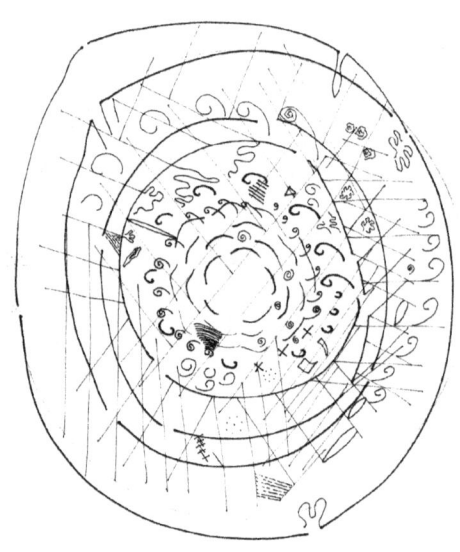

ISBN-13:978-1530749553
ISBN-10:150749557
Email: tamaracpublishers@icloud.com

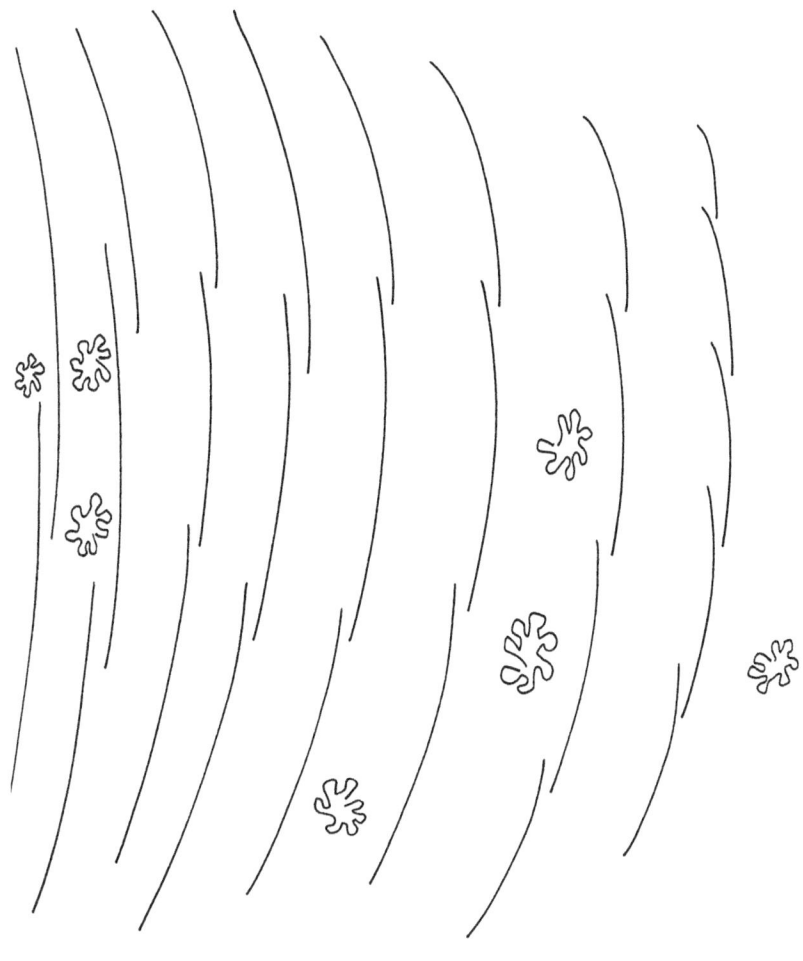

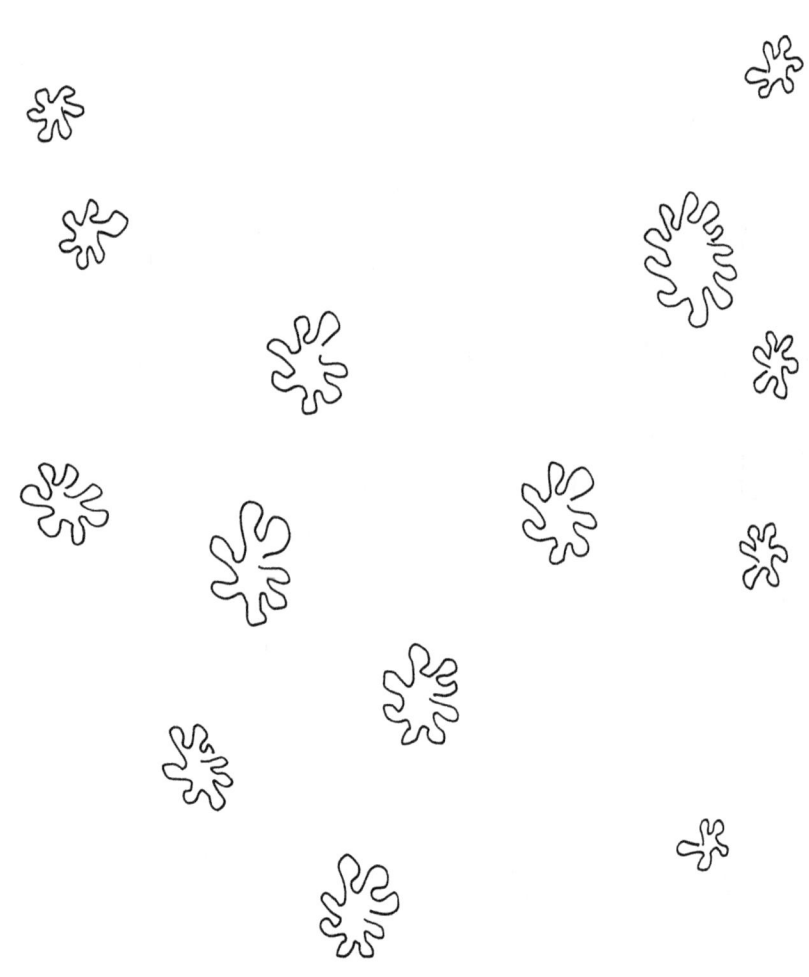

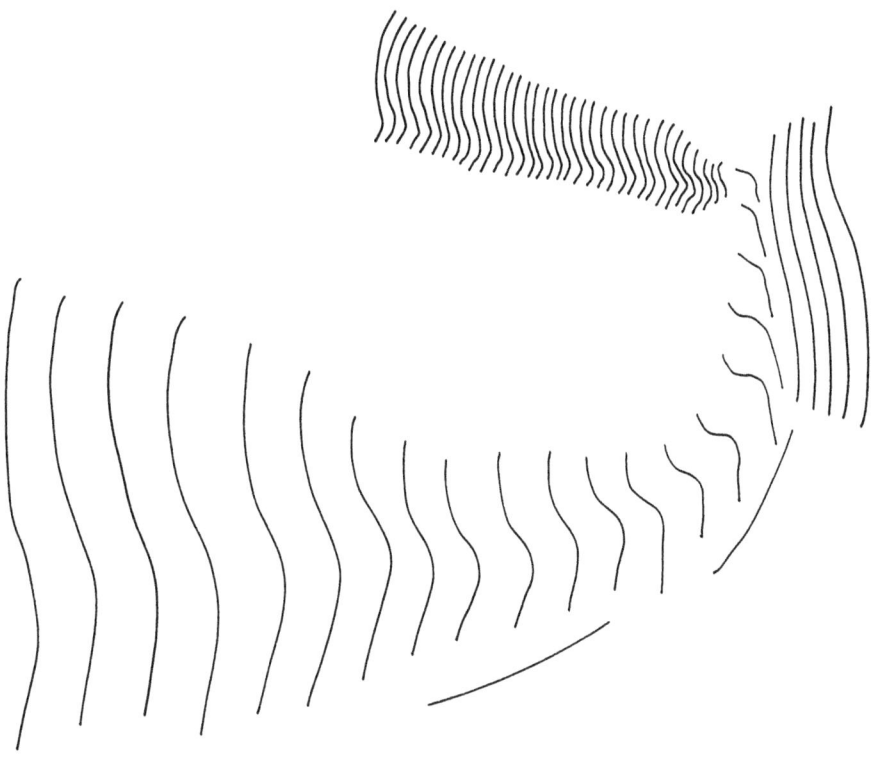

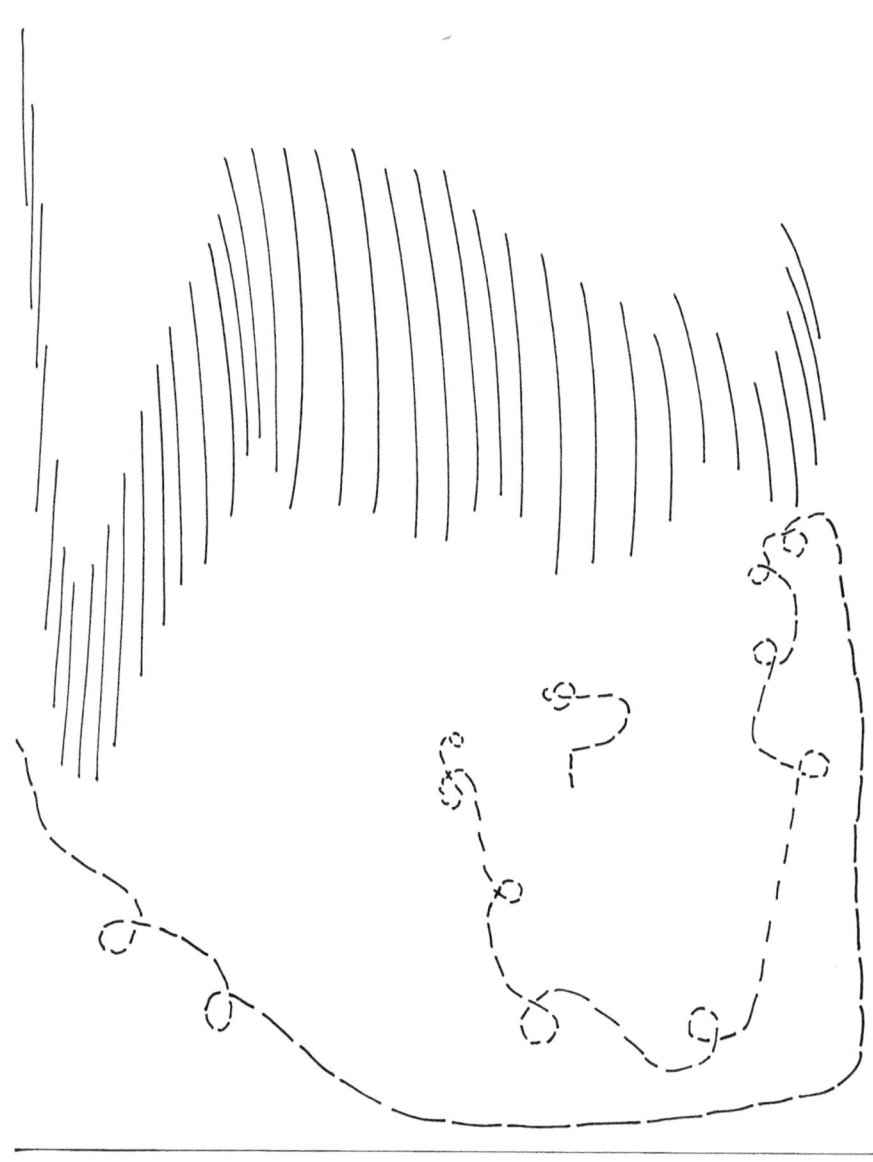

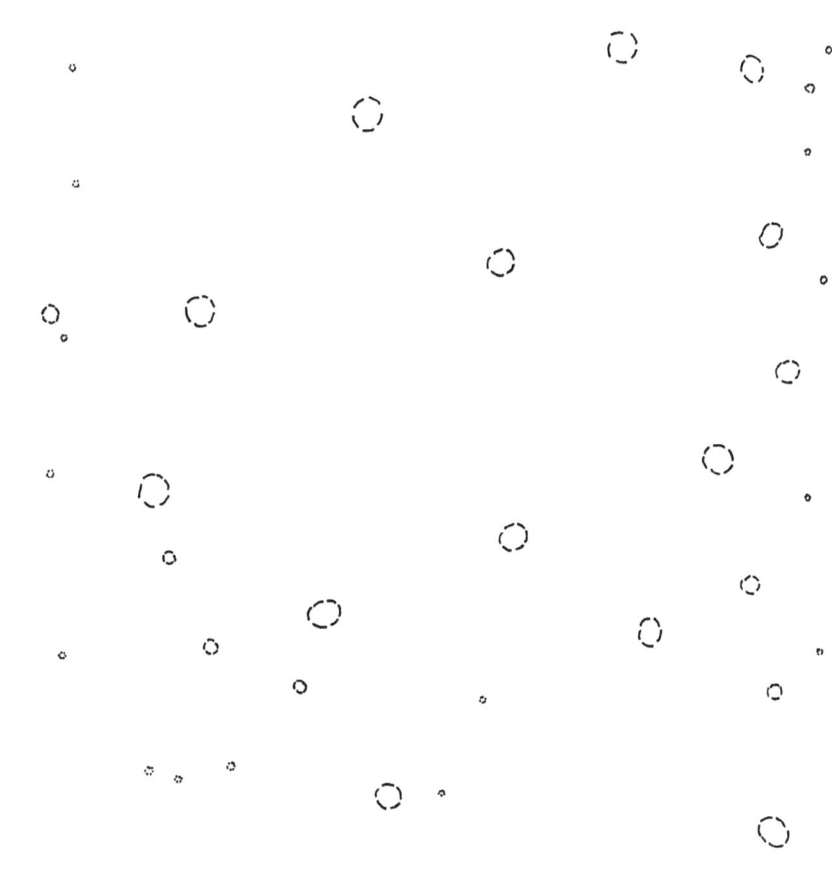

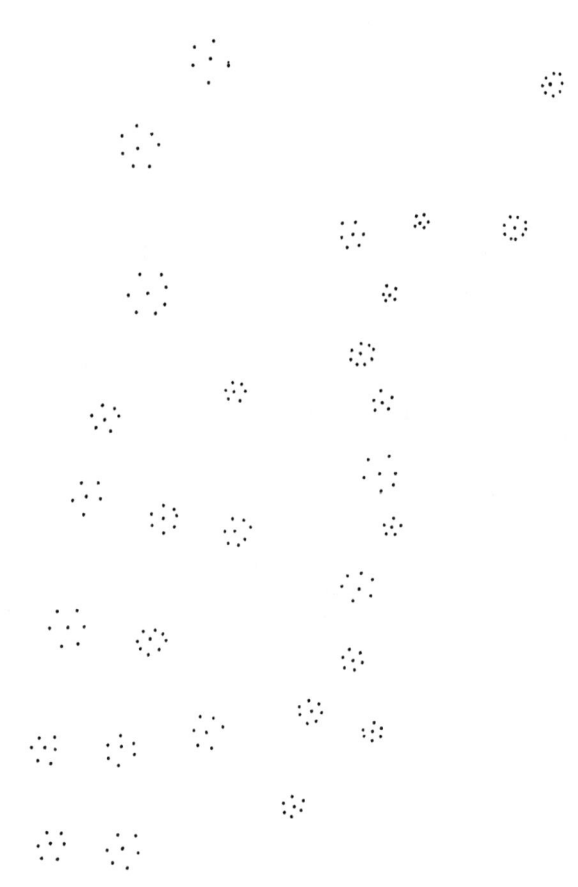

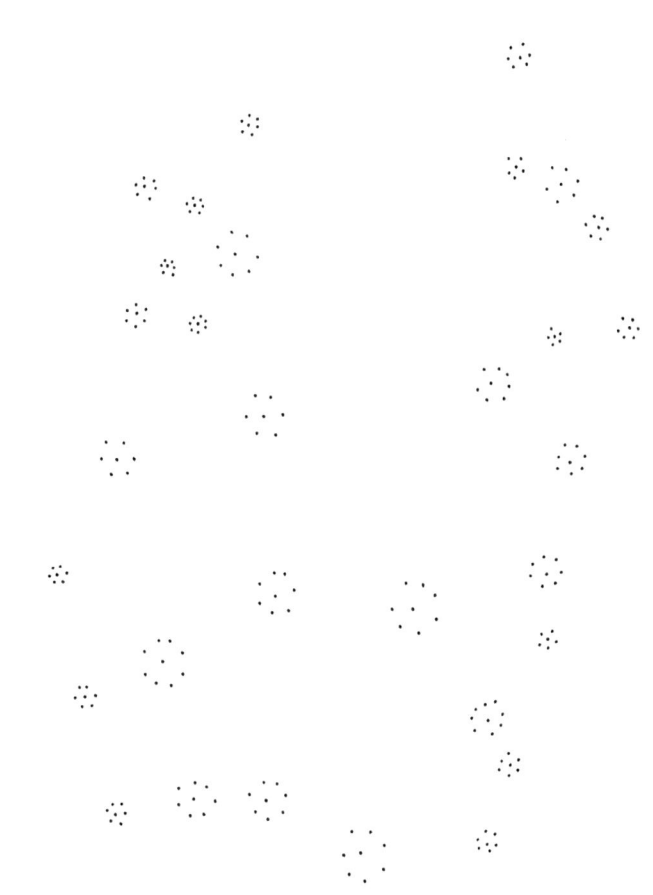

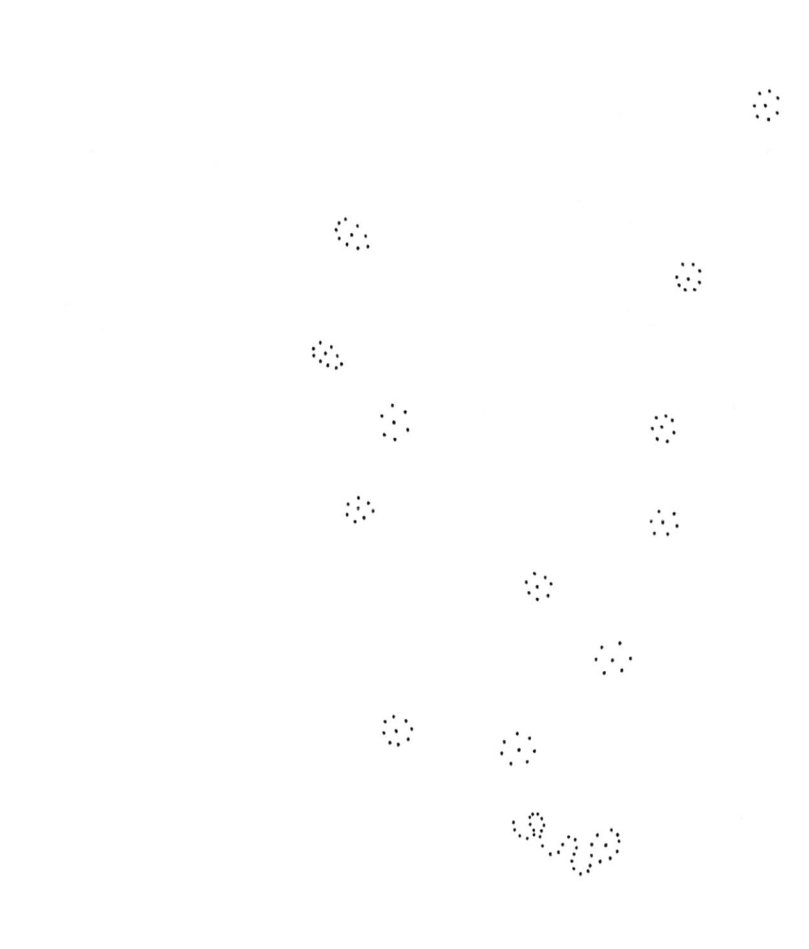

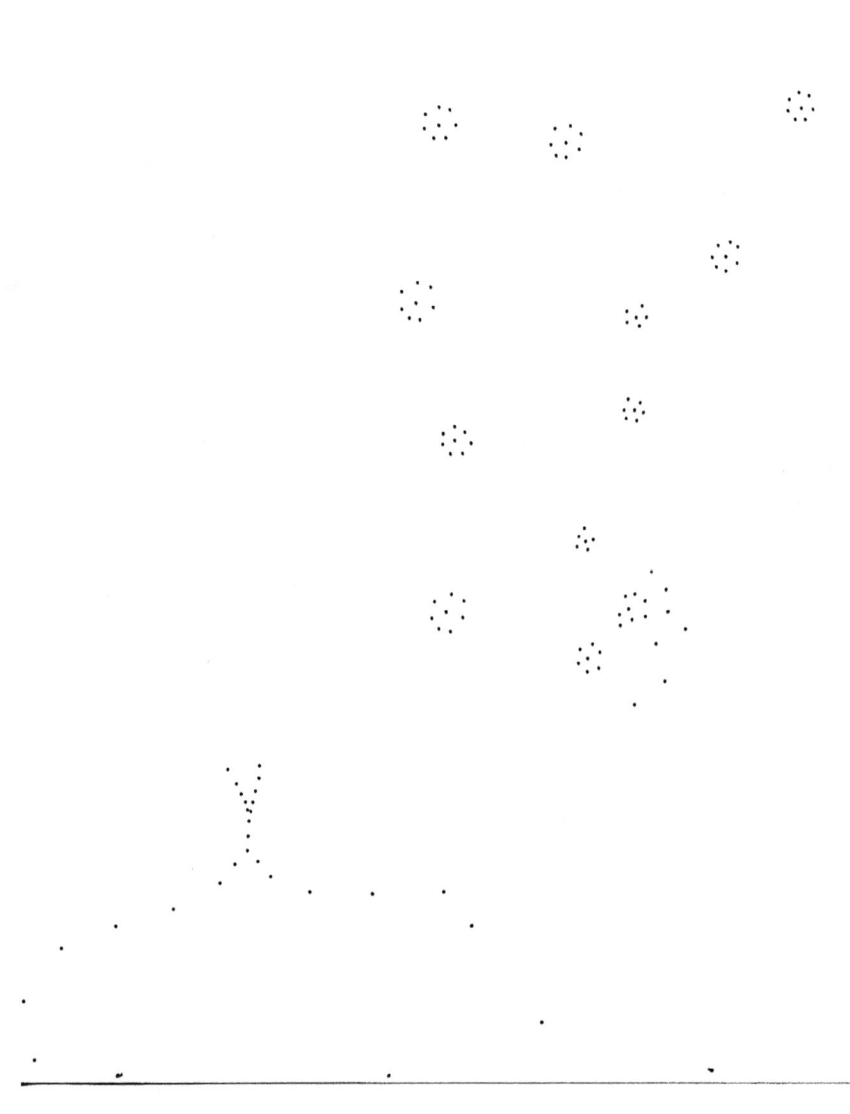

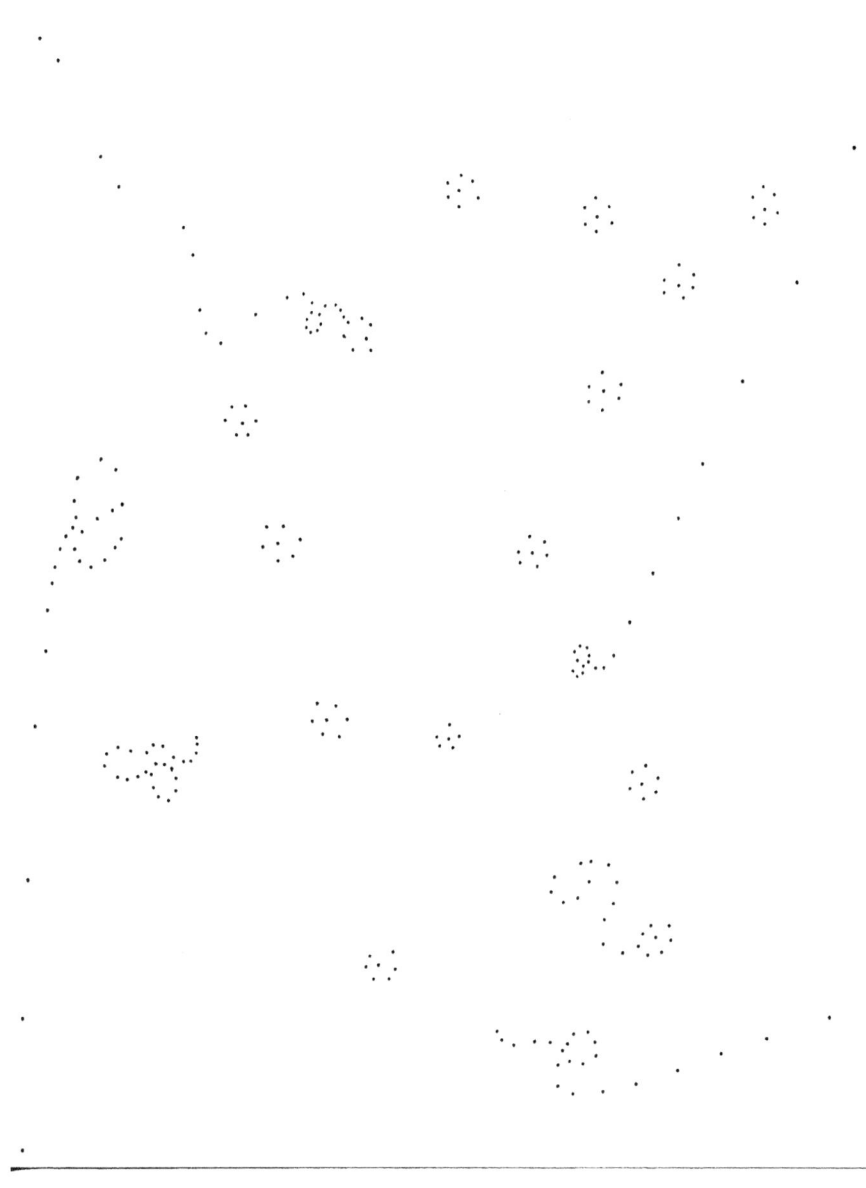

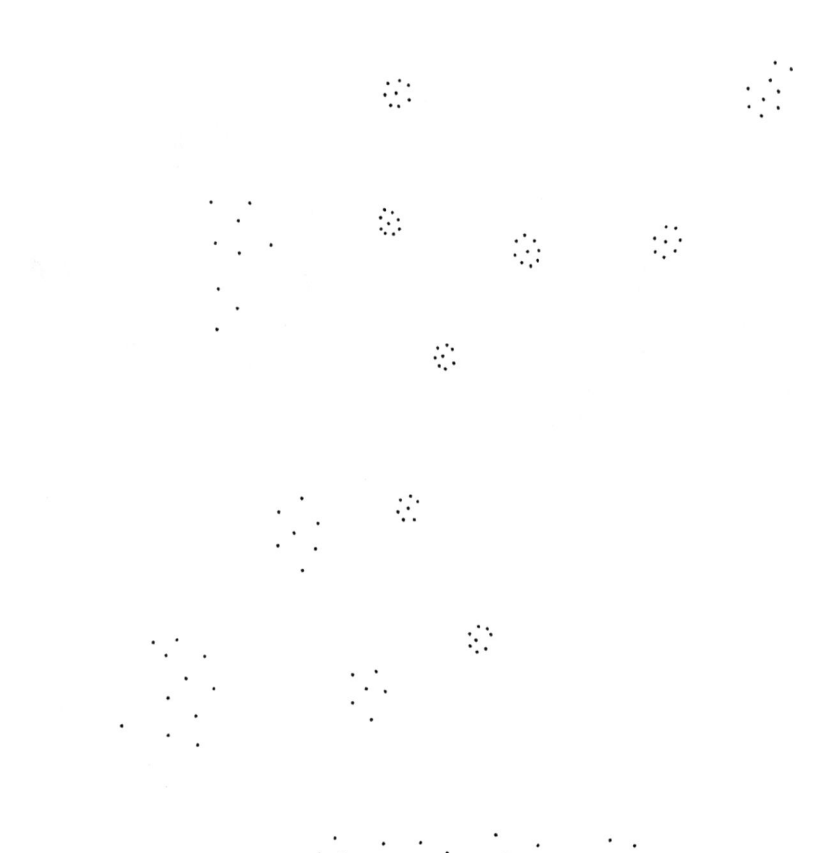

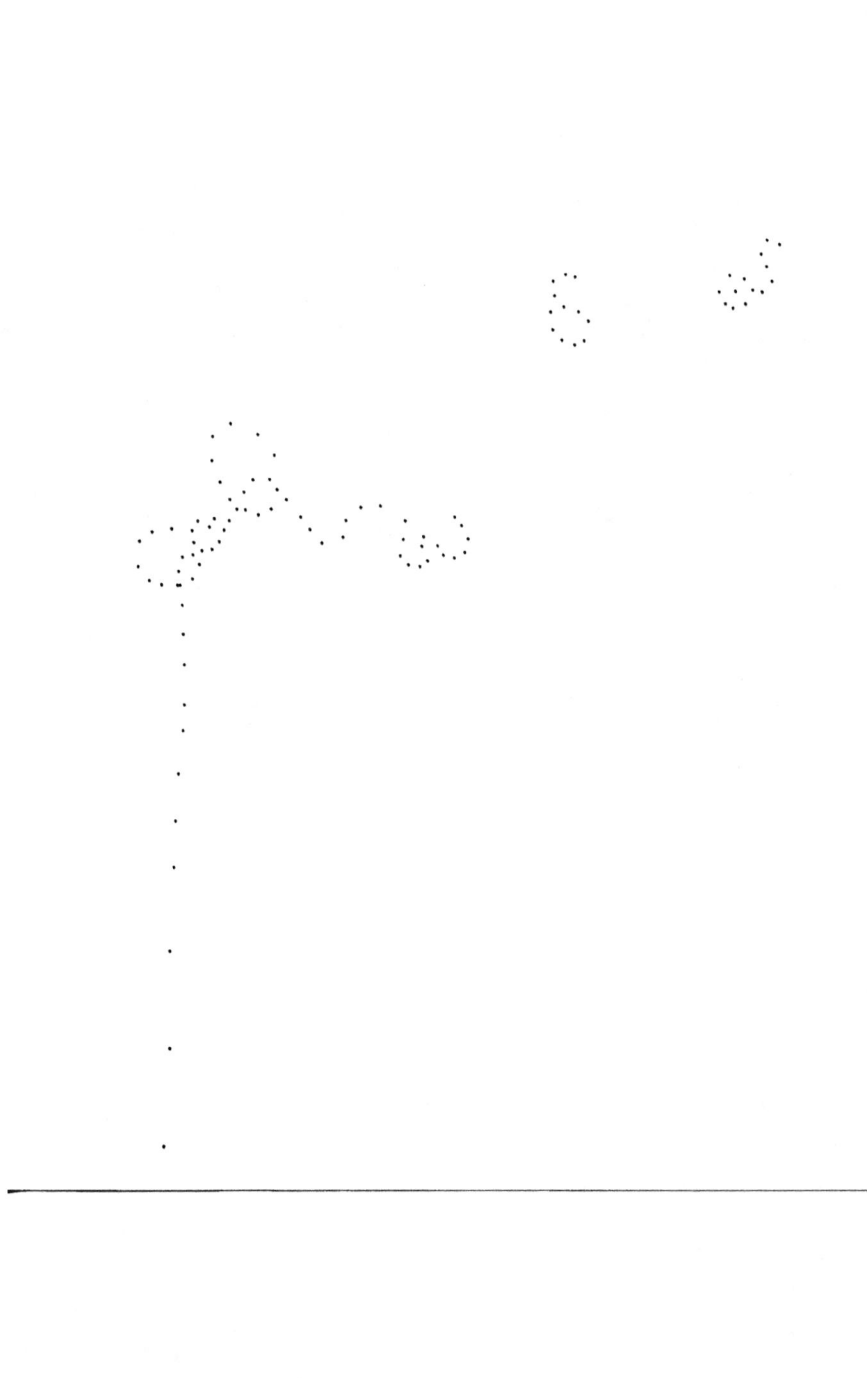

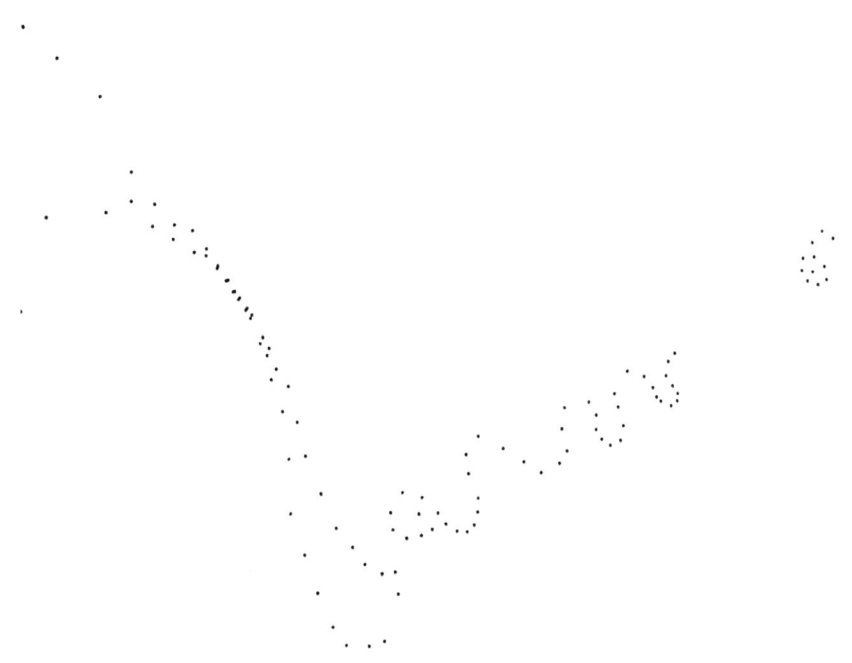

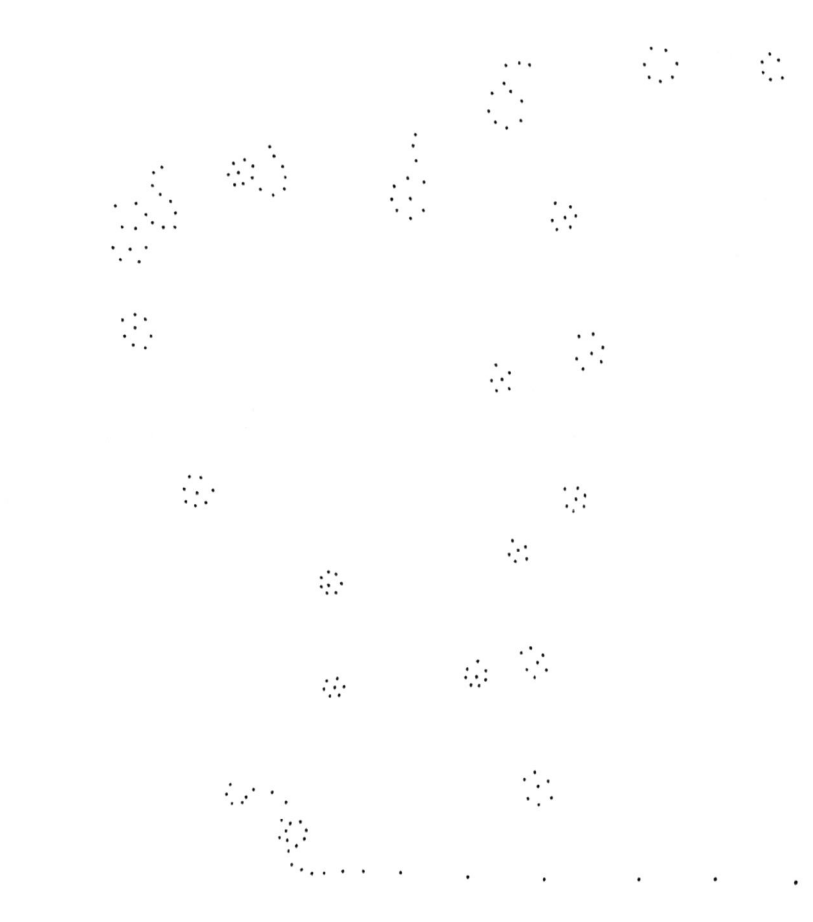

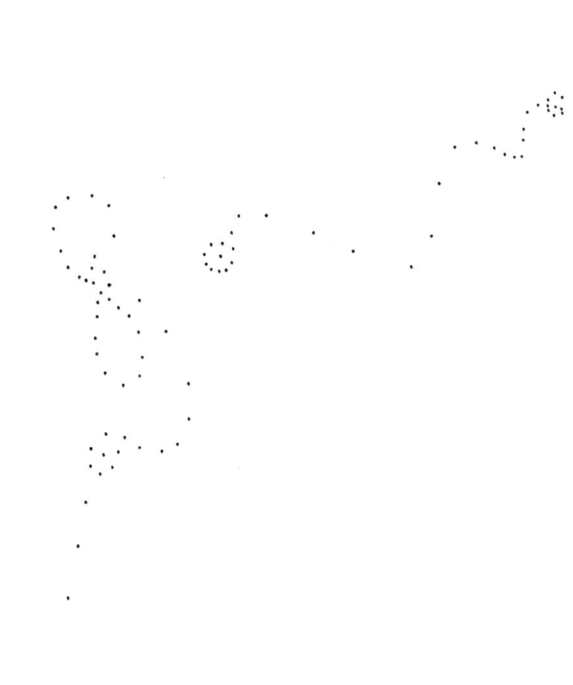

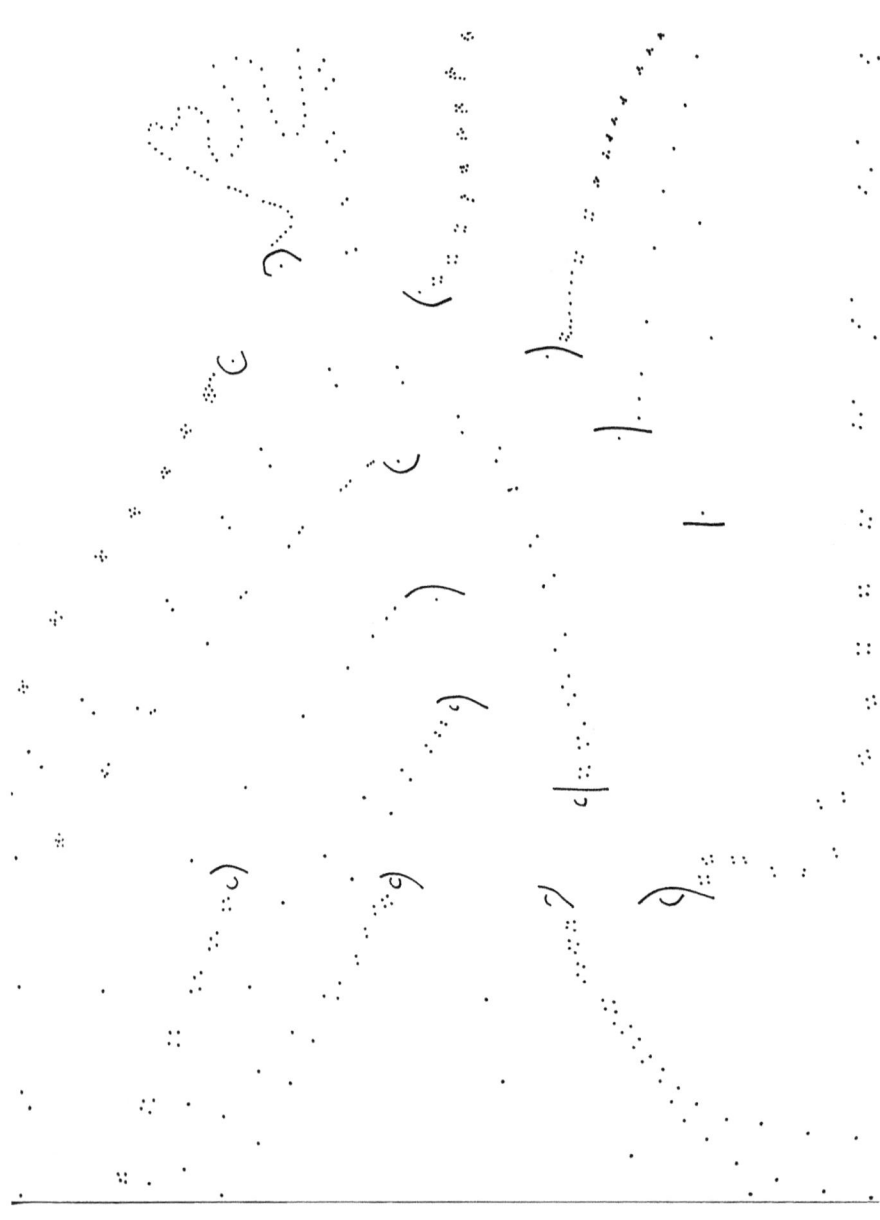

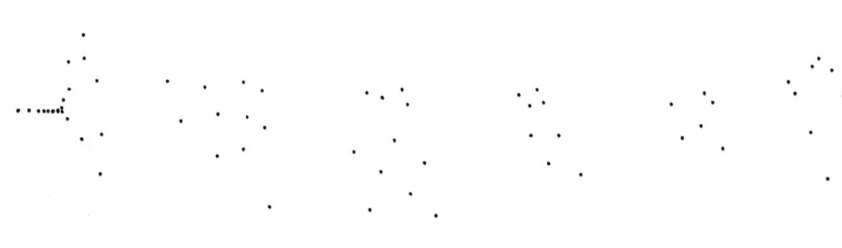

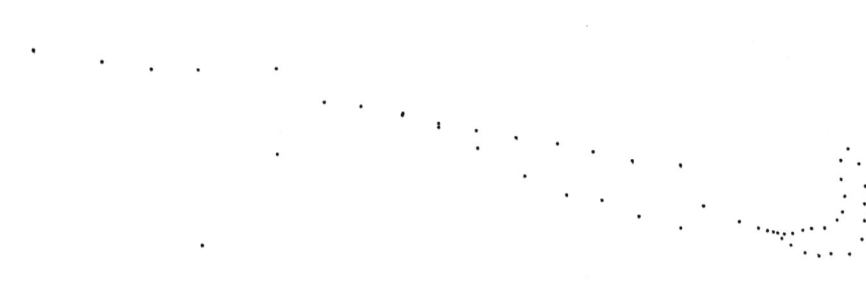

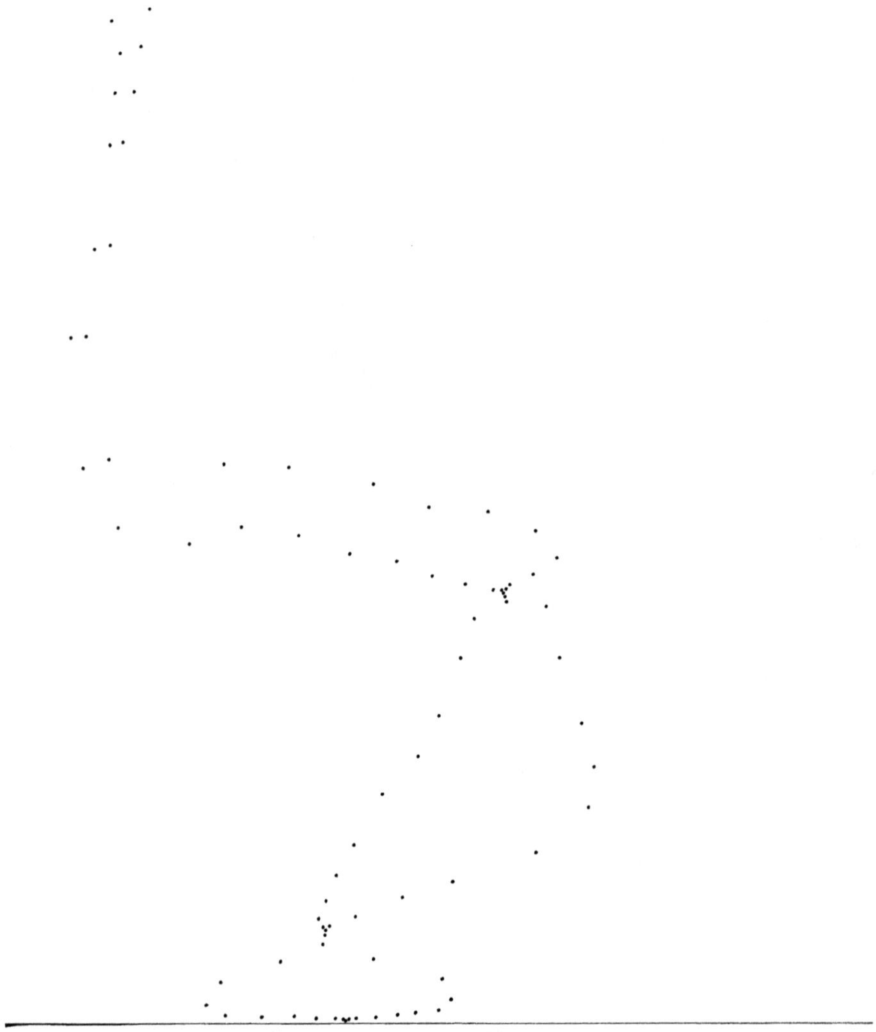

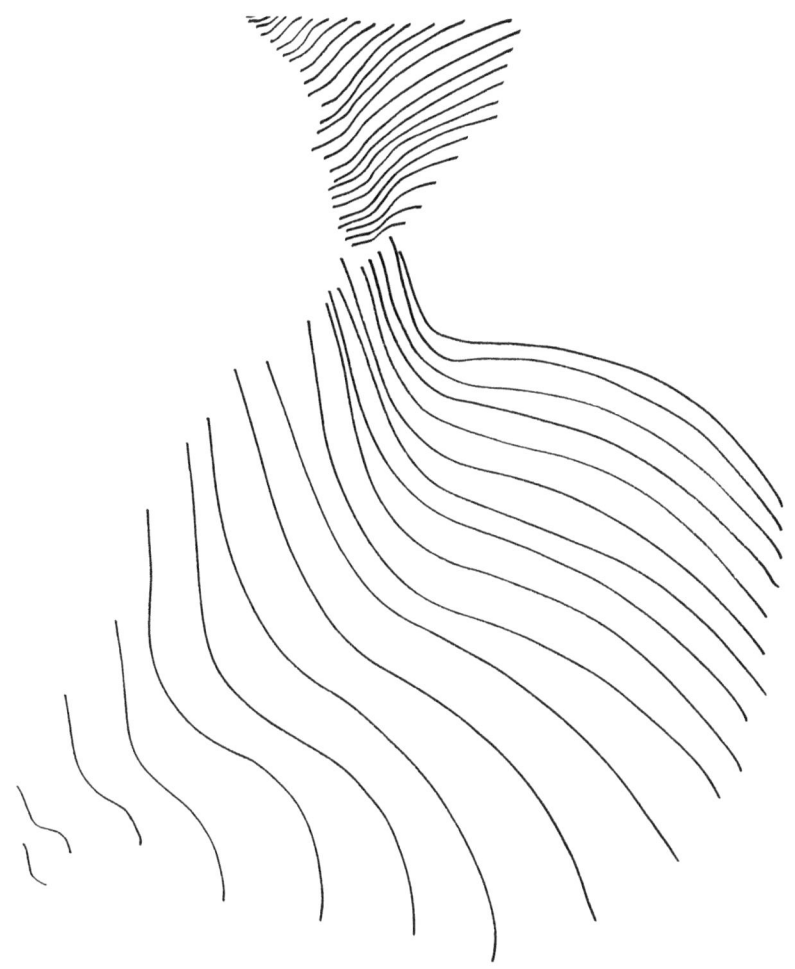

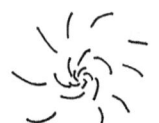

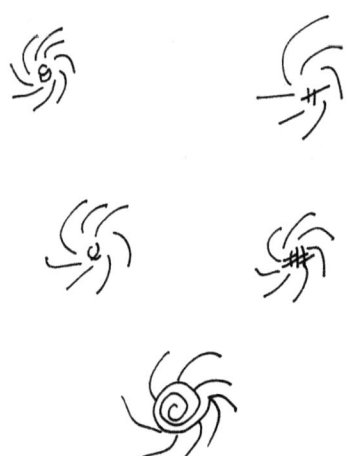

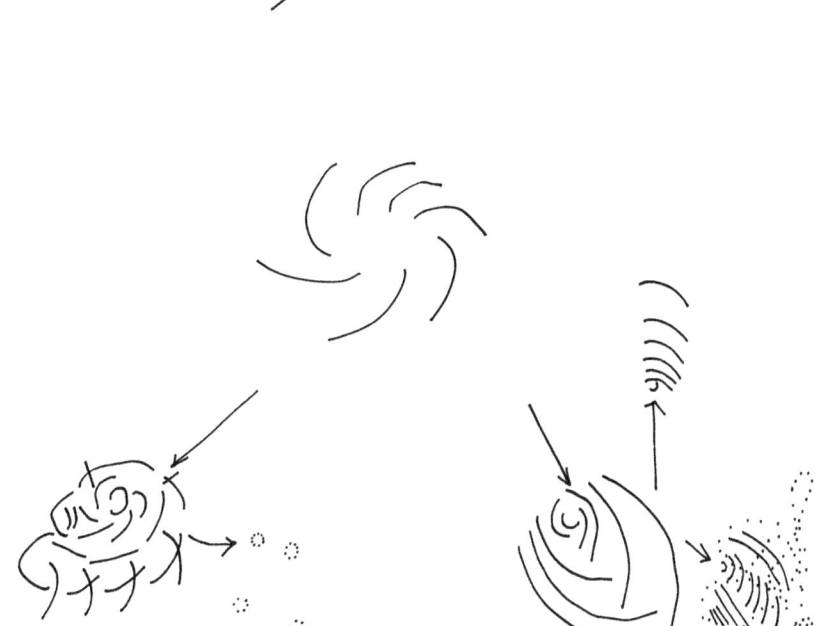

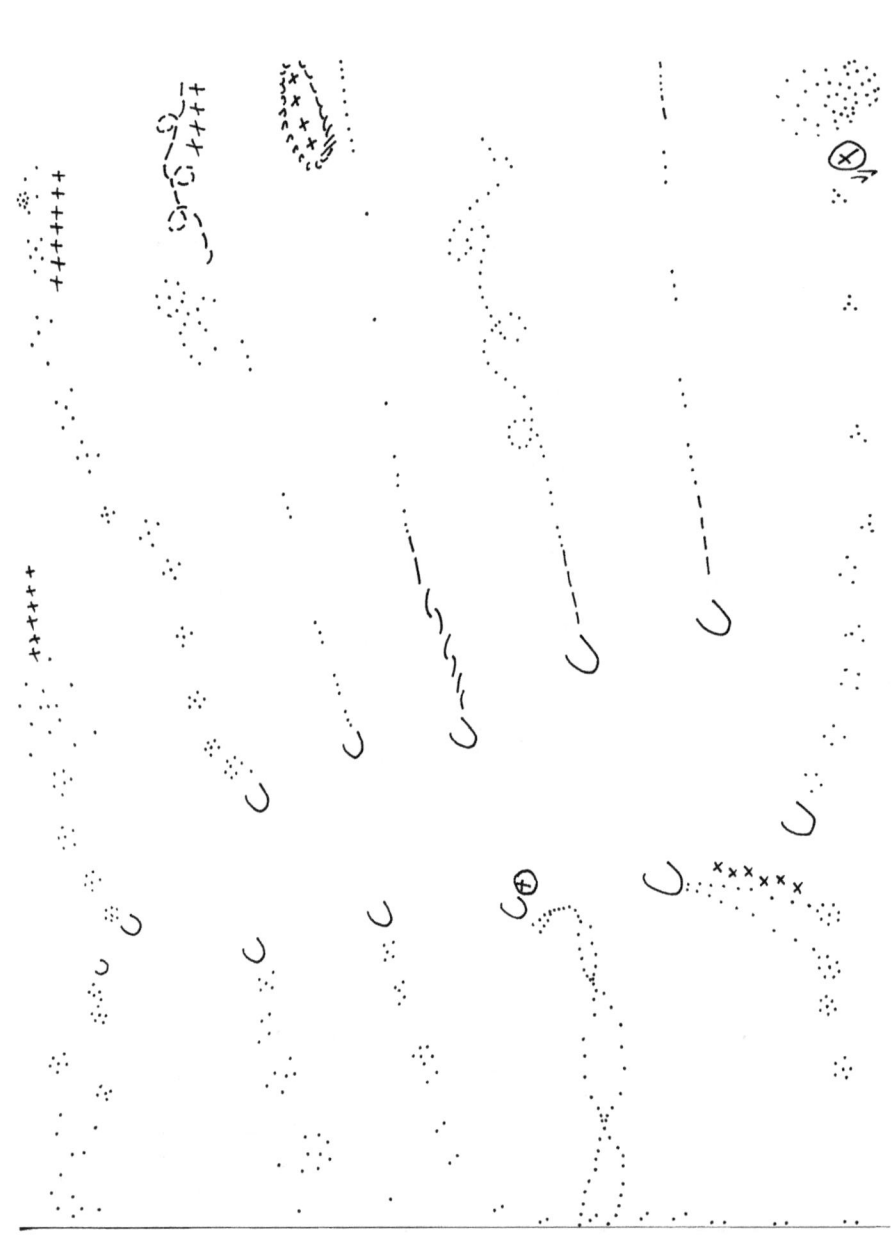

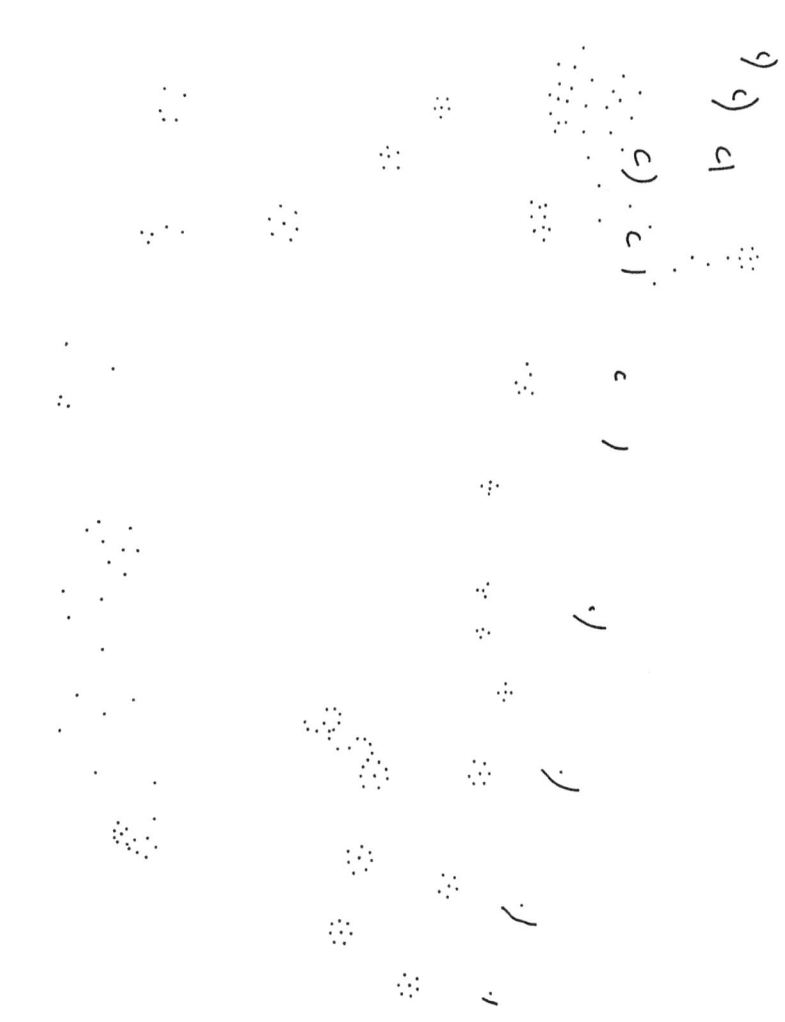

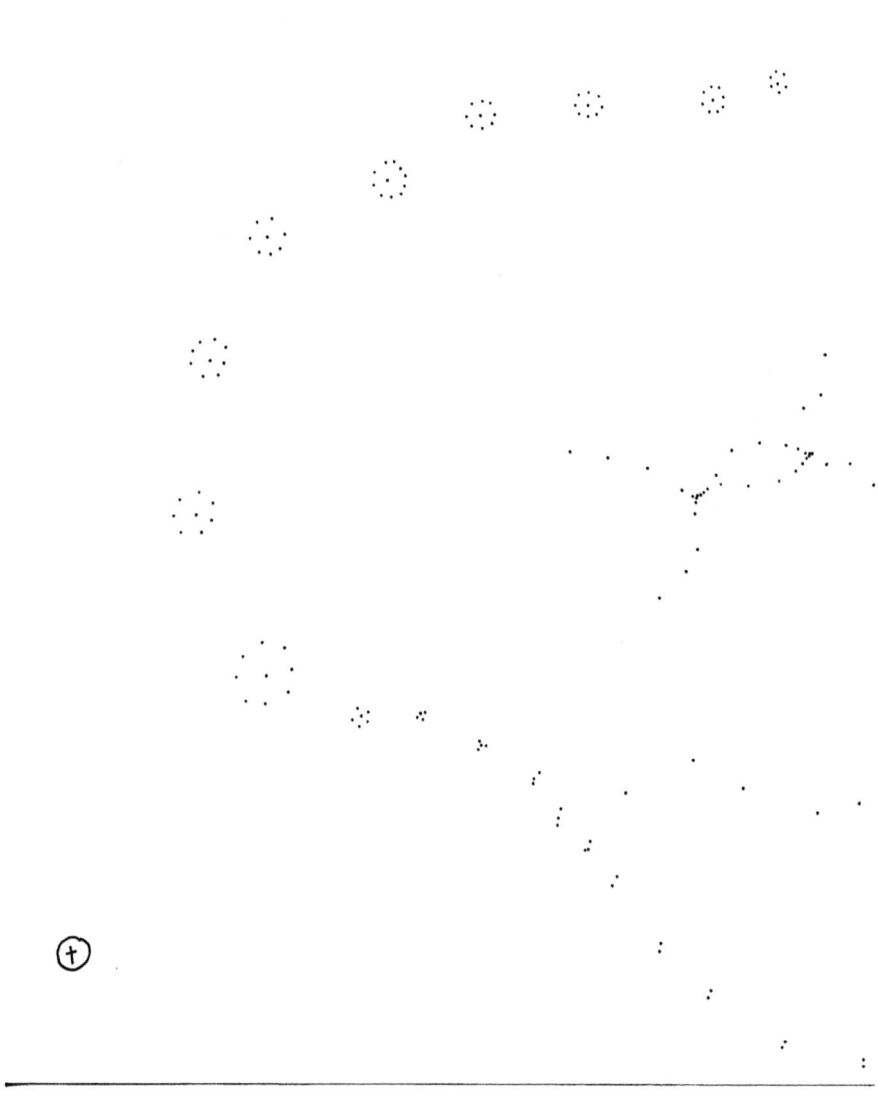

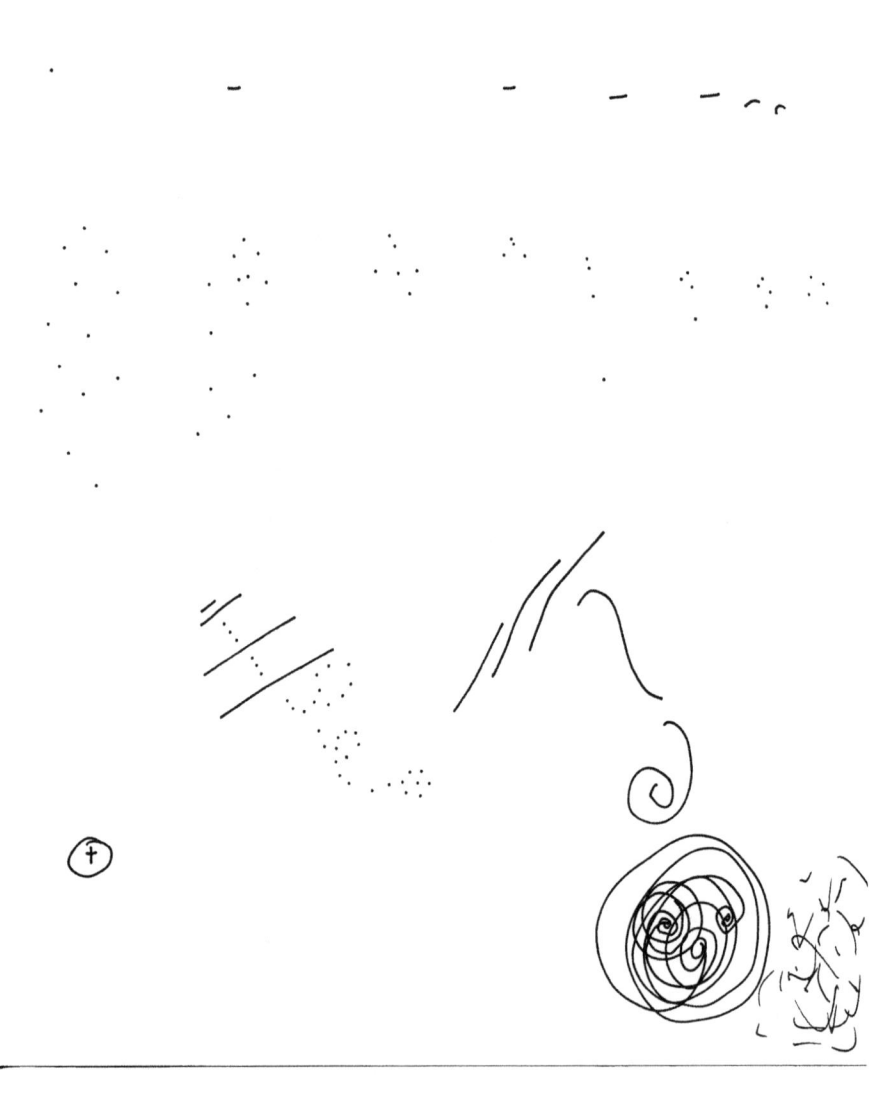

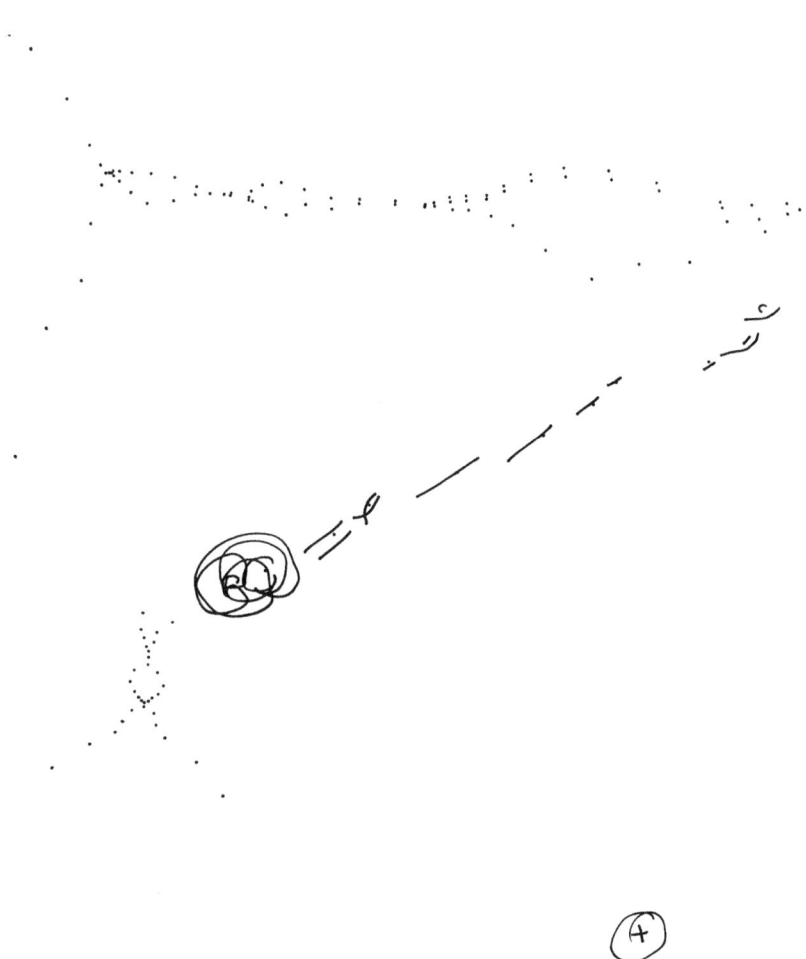

4

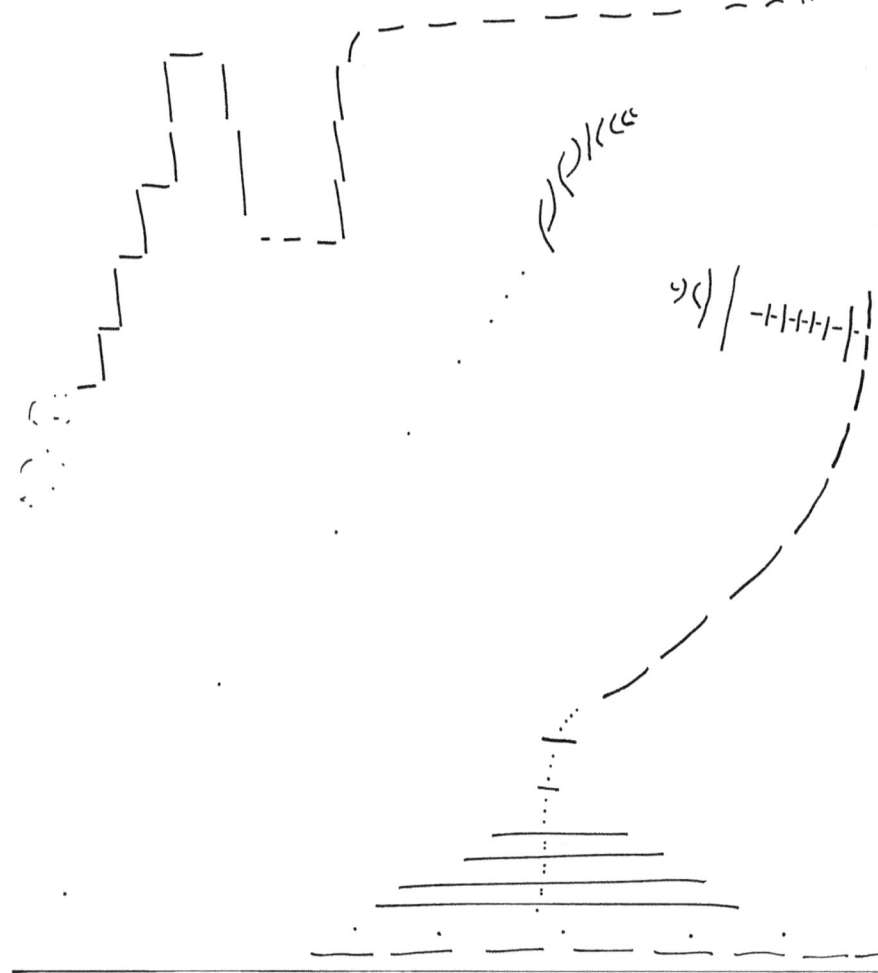

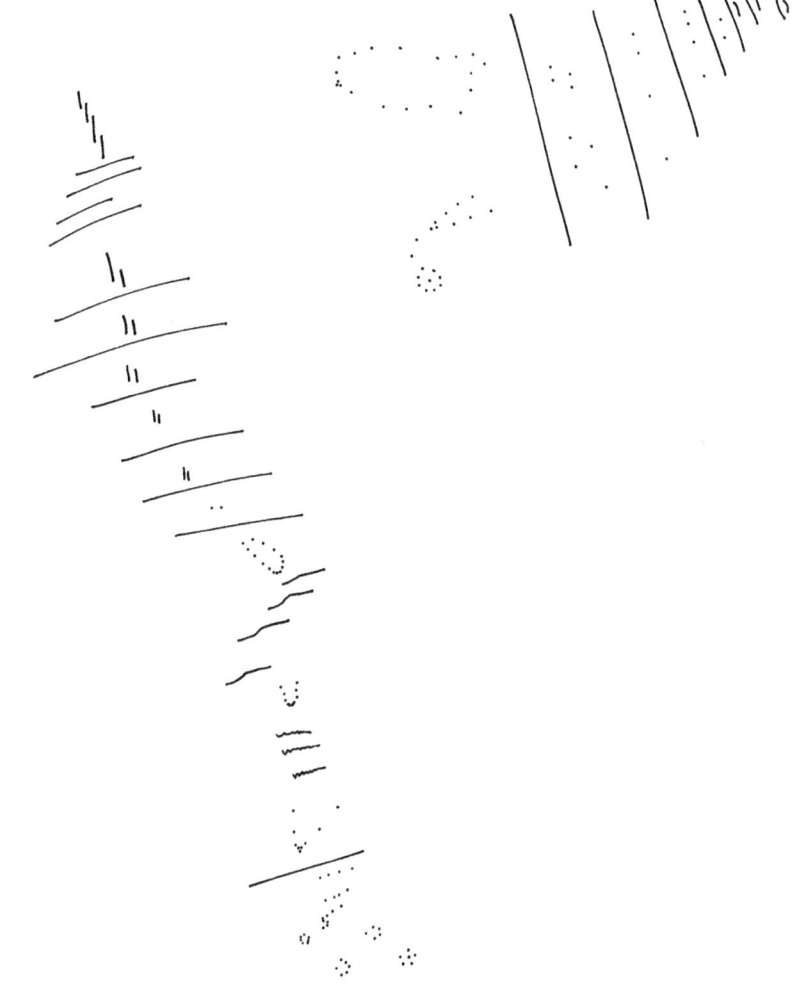

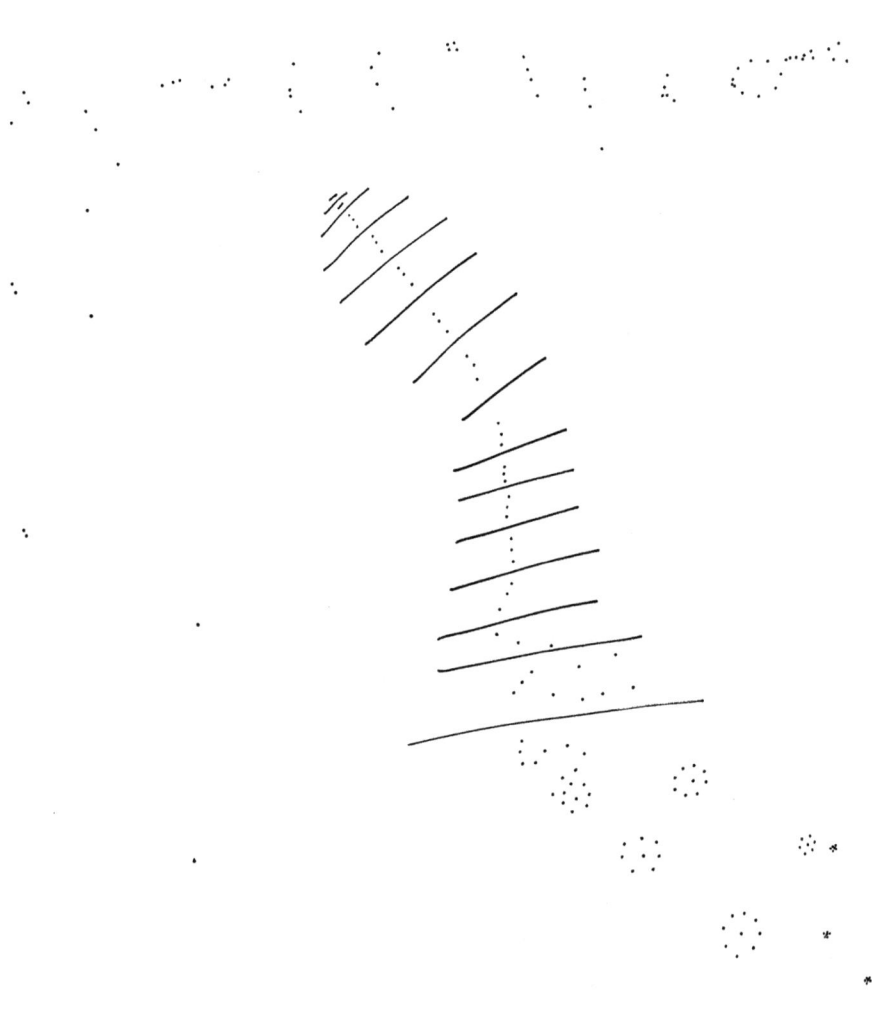

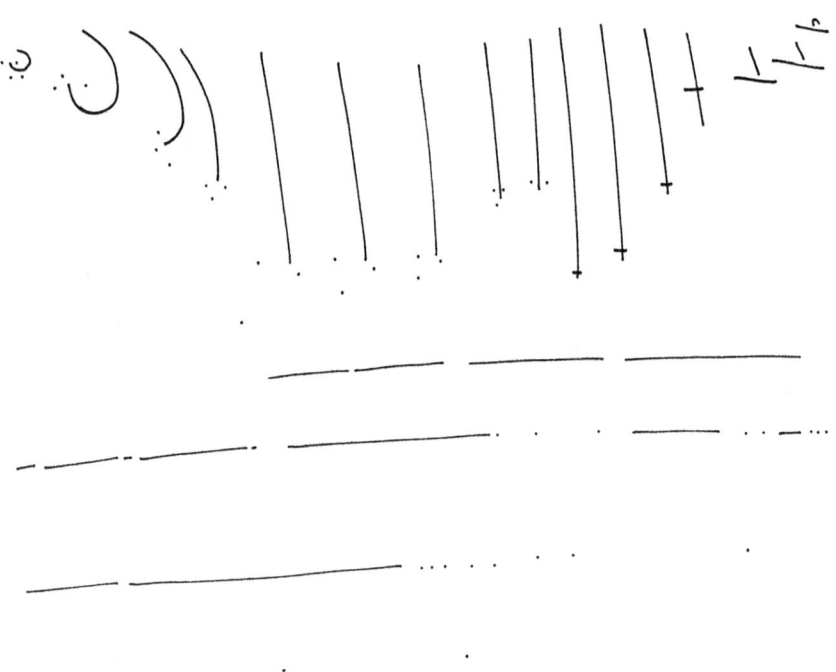

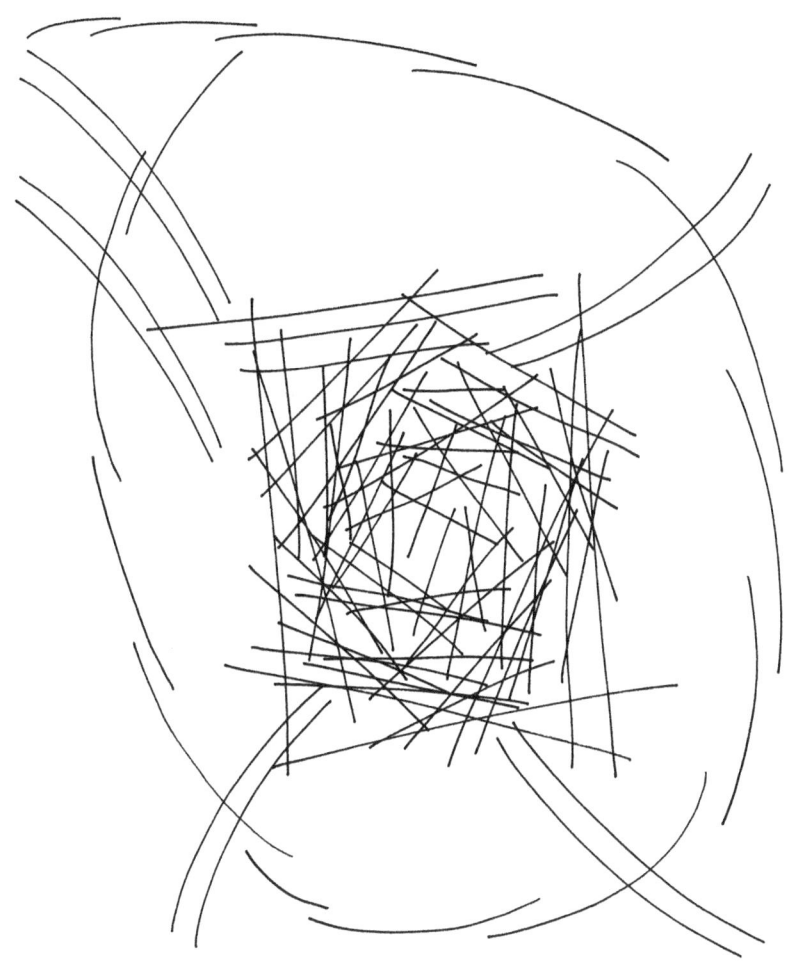